Dr. Sebi Cure for Diabetes

Tasty and Easy Recipes for Detox, Cleanse, and Revitalizing Your Body and Soul Using the Dr. Sebi Food List and Products to Prevent Diabetes

Neal Graham

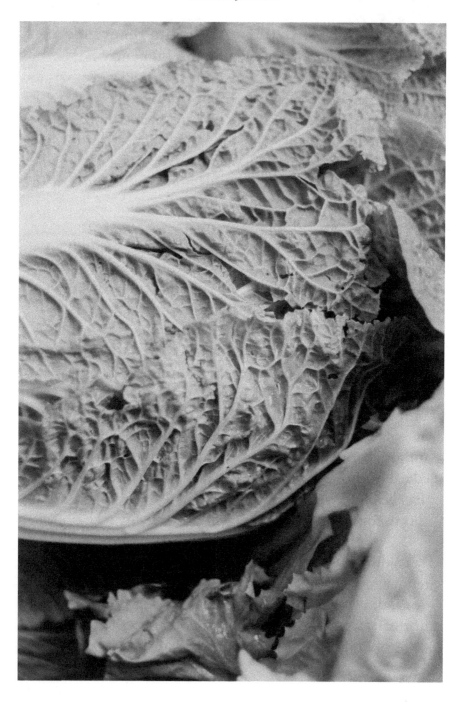

Table of Contents

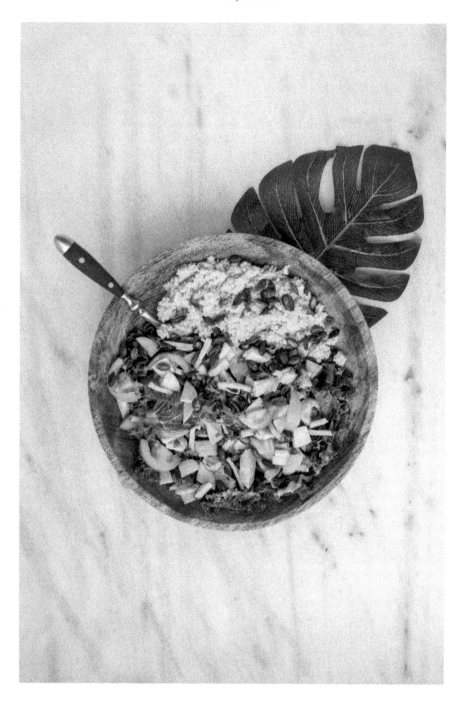

Introduction

Dr. Sebi felt the Western solution to illness was unsuccessful. He held that acidity and mucus — for starters, bacteria, and viruses — induced sickness.

Here are ten strategies to adopt this diet effectively, following these strategies to see results immediately:

1. **Drink water.** Water is probably our body's most famous (after oxygen) resource. Drink between 8-10 glasses of water to keep the body well hydrated (filtered to cleaned).

2. **Avoid acidic drinks like tea, coffee, or soda.** Our body also attempts to regulate acid and alkaline content. There is no need to blink in carbonated beverages as the body refuses carbon dioxide as waste!

3. **Breathe.** Oxygen is the explanation that our body works, and if you provide the body with adequate oxygen, it should perform better. Sit back and enjoy two to five minutes of slow breaths. Nothing is easier than performing Yoga.

4. **Exercise.** Alkaline and the acidic element will also be matched. A little acid (because of muscles) often regulates natural bodywork.

5. **Satiate your urges for a snack by eating vegetables or soaked nuts.** Whenever we are thirsty, we still consume a little fast food. Establish a tradition of consuming fresh vegetables or almonds, even walnuts.

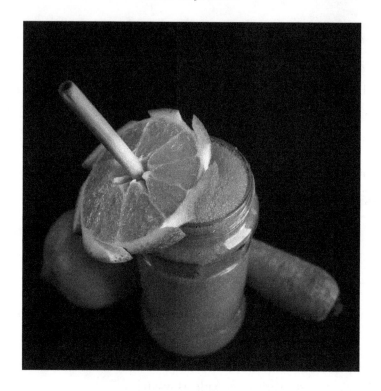

Chapter 1: Doctor Sebi's Food List

When you take a plant diet that has a reduced acid diet, it replaces the animal protein with excess acid. This will promote your kidney because it makes it reduce its work of removing the excess acids present in animal diets.

Besides, bone diseases and many bones associated problems are at times are related to the consumption of some foods that are high in acid. Then, to avoid any bone infections in the body, you must endeavour to eat alkaline diets.

The foods designed by Dr. Sebi are straightforward to acquire around you, and they are cheap and do expensive activities in your body. These foods make you remain lean, clean, and healthy.

Dr. Sebi classified the foods into different categories. These categories are:

- Fruits
- Vegetables
- Alkaline Grains
- Alkaline Sugars

Vegetables

- Cucumber
- Tomatillo
- Turnip greens.
- Wakame

- Onions

- Dandelion greens

- Cherry and plum tomato

- Dulse

- Garbanzo beans

- Izote flower and leaf

- Kale

- Mushrooms except for Shitake

- Arame

- Wild Arugula

- Avocado

- Amaranth

- Bell Pepper

- Chayote

- Hijiki

- Nopales

- Nori

- Zucchini

- Watercress

- Lettuce except for iceberg

- Olives

- Purslane verdolaga

- Squash

- Okra

Fruits

- Apples

- Pears

- Limes

- Mango

- Berries

- Melons

- Prickly pear

- Cherries

- Soursops

- Dates

- Figs

- Grapes

- Prunes

- Raisins

- Papayas

- Bananas

- Cantaloupe

- Currants

- Orange

- Soft jelly coconuts

- Peaches

- Plums

Alkaline Grains

- Spelt

- Fonio

- Quinoa

- Rye

- Kamut

- Tef

- Wild rice

- Amaranth

Alkaline Sugars

- 100% Pure agave syrup extracted from cactus

- Dried date sugar

Diets Designed by Dr. Sebi

The diets designed by Dr. Sebi are essential for the prevention and cure of cancer disease and many other conditions. All sufferers of cancer disease are expected to consume only foods approved by Dr. Sebi, although the diets might be severe for those who are addicted to acidic foods such as rice, soy, beans, alcohol, junks, and many more.

List of Foods to Avoid in Dr. Sebi's Diet

Some foods are disregarded in Dr. Sebi's food list because you must do away with them. Most of these foods could be dangerous for your health, especially for cancer patients.

These foods contain an increasing amount of acidic contents and are not advised to be taken by a cancer patient. Although these foods are suitable for the mouth, they are not good for the body. Dr. Sebi tagged them as forbidden foods. These foods are listed below:

- Alcoholic beverages
- Fish and seafood
- Meat of all kind
- Poultry products
- Colorants and flavours
- Processed foods
- Canned foods and fruits
- Soy and soy products
- Corn

- Genetically modified organism fruits

- Eggs

- Wheat

- Seedless fruits

- Foods with yeast or other components such as baking powder

- Fast foods

- Sugar

- Foods fortified with vitamins and minerals

- Garlic

- Genetically modified organism vegetables

- Dairy foods

Approved Products

While food plays the most significant part in the Dr. Sebi diet, there are products that he recommends you take. Various sites sell Dr. Sebi supplements. Some are more luxurious and expensive than others, but they are all the same things. The goal of the supplements is to provide your body with nutrients that it needs to function correctly. Some supplements are specific to men and women as well, so make sure that you pay attention. Most websites will also provide you with grouped products that offer you everything you need for general health or to heal a specific ailment.

Iron Plus

Iron plus is meant to help purify the entire body. It contains chaparral, which, as we have talked about, is a powerful antioxidant. Iron plus also contains:

- Bugleweed
- Palo guaco
- Hombre grande
- Blue vervain
- Chaparral
- Elderberry

Green Food

This is a multi-mineral supplement that is made up of herbs from Africa and offers chlorophyll-rich food that nourished the body. It contains ortiga, which is well known as an anti-inflammatory. It can also help with gout, rheumatism, influenza, hemorrhage, cardiovascular system, locomotor system disorders, gastrointestinal tract disorders, urinary tract infections, and kidney disorders. It is also great at helping poor circulation and purifying the blood. Ortiga has also been used to improve the symptoms of hay fever. Green food contains:

- Bladderwrack
- Nopal
- Tila
- Nettle

Bromide Plus Powder/Bromide Plus Capsules

This is meant to help your thyroid gland and bones. It is excellent for people who suffer from dysentery, respiratory issues, pulmonary illnesses, and bad breath. It is a natural diuretic, improves the digestive system, regulates the bowels, and suppresses the appetite. It contains bladderwrack, which is a seaweed that lives in the Baltic Sea, Atlantic Ocean, and the Pacific Ocean. It is one of the sources of iodine. It is full of mannitol, alginic, potassium, bromine, and beta-carotene. It contains bladderwrack and Irish sea moss.

Bio Ferro Tonic/Bio Ferro Capsules

Bio Ferro contains the right ingredients to purify and nourish the blood. It includes a yellow dock root, which is an herb that acts as a digestive bitter to help improve digestion. It is a detoxifier and blood purifier and especially helps the liver. Yellow dock root also helps the metabolism of fats and stimulates bile production. It can also help with bowel movements and get rid of waste lingering in the intestinal tract. It will also increase urination. Bio Ferro contains:

- Cocolmeca
- Yellow dock root
- Burdock root
- Chaparral
- Elderberry

Bio ferro capsules work the same way as the tonic. They have slightly different ingredients even though they do the same thing. The capsules contain:

- Yellow dock root

- Nopal
- Nettle
- Burdock root
- Chaparral

Banju

The banju tonic is made from potent ingredients to make a tonic that helps to stimulate the central nervous system and brain. It contains:

- Bugleweed
- Valerian root
- Burdock root
- Blue vervain
- Elderberry

Body Care

Uterine Oil and Wash

As you can presumption by the name, this is meant for women. This helps to cleanse and restore the flora and fauna of the vagina. The red clover in the wash acts as a blood purifier, improves circulation, and acts as an expectorant. It also contains isoflavones and flavonoids, which help to produce estrogen. Red clover is excellent at treating conditions that are associated with menopause. The ingredients in the wash include:

- Red clover
- Sage
- Arnica
- Lupulo

Tooth Powder

This is a natural powder that you can use as a toothpaste that will help stop gum disease and tooth decay. It contains Encino and myrrh gum powder.

Hair Food Oil

This is meant to nourish the scalp and hair. It is gentle on the skin so that it can be used every day. It helps stimulate hair growth. It contains:

- French vanilla

- Coconut oil

- Batana oil

- Olive oil

Eyewash

This product naturally cleanses and nourishes the eye. It contains the only eyebright, which is commonly used to help treat many different eye diseases. It can also aid to reduce the inflammation in the eye caused by conjunctivitis and blepharitis.

Eva Salve

This salve is meant to tone and nourish the skin. The unique combination of ingredients in eva salve provides natural minerals the skin needs like potassium phosphate, fluorine, and calcium, which your skin needs to maintain elasticity. It also contains sage which is a powerful antioxidant that helps to fight off free radical damage. Eva salve contains:

- Manzo

- Eucalyptus

- Sage
- Arnica
- Olive oil
- Lily of the valley
- Nopal
- Shea butter
- Estro

Herbal Teas

- Stomach relief tea
- Stress relief tea
- Immune support tea
- Energy booster tea
- Cold and cough tea
- Blood pressure balance tea

Foods to Avoid

Any foods that are not covered in the Dr. Sebi vitamins manual aren't accredited, which includes:

- Canned fruit or vegetables
- Seedless fruit
- Eggs
- Dairy
- Fish
- Red meat

- Rooster

- Soy products

- Processed meals, including take-out or eating place meals

- Fortified ingredients

- Wheat

- Sugar (except date sugar and agave syrup)

- Alcohol

- Yeast or foods rose with yeast

- Meals made with baking powder

Furthermore, many greens, grains, nuts, and seeds are banned on the diet. Only foods indexed inside the guide can be eaten. The food regimen limits any food this is processed, animal-primarily based, or made with leavening.

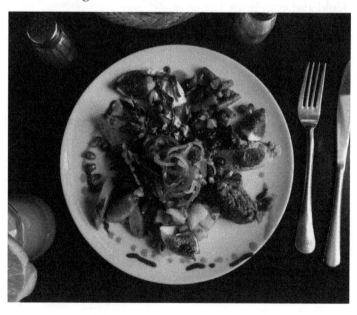

Chapter 2: How to Follow the Diet

Rules to Follow

To follow Dr. Sebi's diet, you need to strictly adhere to his rules, which are present on his website. Here is a list of his guidelines below:

1. Do not eat or drink any product or ingredient not mentioned in the approved list for the diet. It is not recommended and should never be consumed when following the diet.

2. You have to drink almost one gallon (or more than three liters) of water every day. It is recommended to drink spring water.

3. You have to take Dr. Sebi's mixtures or products one hour before consuming your medications.

4. You can take any of Dr. Sebi's mixtures/products together without any worry.

5. You need to follow the nutritional guidelines stringently and punctually take Dr. Sebi's mixtures/products daily.

6. You are not allowed to consume any animal-based food or hybrid products.

7. You are not allowed to consume alcohol or any kind of dairy product.

8. You are not allowed to consume wheat, only natural growing grains as listed in the nutritional guide

9. The grains mentioned in the nutritional guide can be available in different forms, like pasta and bread, in different health food stores. You can consume them.

10. Do not use fruits from cans; also, seedless fruits are not recommended for consumption.

11. You are not allowed to use a microwave to reheat your meals.

How to Prepare the Body

It should be clear that it is a restrictive diet low in calories. Many people believe that because of this reason, it cannot be used as a standard way to lose weight as it puts too much stress on the body of a new dieter. Because it is low in calories and an intensive diet, weight loss can be seen, but the person needs to assess whether they are capable of handling a low caloric diet. Being too ambitious with this diet might turn fatal, so if you want to try the diet, be careful!

This diet has been suggested to be followed throughout one's entire life, which might not be possible for a new dieter. With any diet, if you start cutting foods strongly and then revert to your old routine of eating unhealthy meals, the chances are that the weight loss and benefits you see will get reversed. This is a risk in this diet as well. When starting, set reasonable goals and don't go too strongly. Let your body first get used to it and then start setting up more ambitious goals.

Meal Plan

Starting the diet can be daunting, so here is a list of meal ideas that you can copy from. For the first few days, follow it so that you get used to the diet.

Breakfast

1. Banana pancakes with agave syrup (more than one is recommended).

2. A strawberry and banana smoothie with added hemp seeds and water.

3. Cooked quinoa with coconut milk (pure) and agave syrup for sweetness (add a fruit of your choice as well).

Lunch

1. A salad made up of kale, tomatoes, onions, avocados, and chickpeas with olive oil and dressing of herbs.

2. A pizza made with spelt flour, Brazil nut cheese topped with different vegetables like tomatoes, etc.

3. A pasta made of spelt with different vegetables, and lime and olive oil dressings.

Evening Snack

1. A smoothie made by cucumbers, kale, a few pieces of ginger, and one or two apples.

2. Herbal tea accompanied by the fruit of your choice.

3. Blueberry muffins made by spelt and teff flour, coconut milk (pure), agave syrup, and blueberries.

Dinner

1. A wild rice stir-fry with vegetables of your choice.

2. A burger made up of spelt flour bread; tomatoes, onions, and kale as vegetables; and a chickpea patty.

3. Thick vegetable soup made up of zucchini, mushrooms, peppers, spices, sea salt, onions, and seaweed powder.

Drink Water

Smoothies are a drink, and by drinking them, you are ultimately fulfilling your water intake for the day. Dr. Sebi's diet requires you to drink one gallon of water daily, but that can be difficult. Dehydration is a serious problem that can lead to anxiety. To prevent that, you need to drink lots of water, which the smoothie diet helps you with.

What You Should Not Eat

Foods that are not listed in the nutritional guide are not allowed to be consumed. Some examples of such foods are given below:

1. Any canned product, be it fruits or vegetables, listed in the nutritional guide

2. Seedless fruits like grapes

3. Eggs

4. Any type of dairy product

5. Fish

6. Any type of poultry

7. Red meat

8. Soy products

9. Processed foods

10. Restaurant foods and delivered foods

11. Hybrid and fortified foods

12. Wheat

13. White sugar

14. Alcohol

15. Yeast and its products

16. Baking powder

Some other foods and ingredients have been cut off. You only need to follow the nutritional guide to know what you have to eat.

A 7-Day Alkaline Meal Plan

Among the diverse body parts, the liver is among one of the significant organs, for it has considerable capacity in body detoxification. Through this body detoxification, synthetics and other outside substances like poisons and even defecation, pee, and sweat are expelled from the body. These substances originate from the unsafe nourishments that we eat like handled and non-regular rich nourishments, liquor drinks that we devour, cigarettes that we smoke, and even drugs that we expend for anti-infection treatment and hormone elective drugs. These substances are the ones that our bodies attempt to take out every day.

When there are many harming materials inside the body, the liver needs to keep keeping up until its ability runs out. When this is dismissed, vast amounts of poisons can be gathered in the body and will cause many body issues and diseases. To anticipate this and keep up excellent health, we should experience a detoxification diet and take significant consideration of our liver.

A liver detoxification plan can be completed either on a three-day, seven-day, or twenty-one-day program. This depends on a firm focus on a diet with unprocessed and natural foods grown from the ground, entire grains, and water cure with enough measure of water or liquid other option. Nourishments that are wealthy in fat or sugar, caffeine, liquor drinks, unnatural and human-made nourishment, drugs, and low-quality nourishments would all be able to must be put to a stop, at any rate, seven days before the diet plan.

One to Three Days. This is the period to start your fluid diet plan where you need to drink around ten to twelve glasses of water ordinarily alongside frequently crushed lime juice. Even though it can indeed be challenging to execute this diet because of the weariness and slightness, light exercise can be included as a request to affix the method of flushing the poisons out of the body. Additionally, you should shun taking in any sort of milk or dairy item.

Four to Six Days. Fresh organic products, vegetables, and entire grains can be expended like celery, apples, carrots, oranges, which would all be able to be blended into one juice. The juice can incorporate your selection of leafy foods. Even though healthy nourishments are devoured, there are as yet liquid choices, for example, natural teas for around a few cups every day. Concerning suppers, they can incorporate cut and bubbled vegetables like celery, carrots, broccoli, and spinach. Besides, you can likewise utilize soups that can be taken in at regular intervals.

Seven Days. Along with the leafy foods, the liquids are expended together. They would all be able to be arranged by having them crude or steamed. Additionally, you can consume rosemary tea and dandelion options, which can be useful for this period.

You can generally change the sorts of foods grown from the ground that you will use as long as you oblige the strategy. When the seventh day is a doe, you can participate in the typical diet; finally, however, there is still a restriction on liquor consumption for around one entire week after the detoxification diet. You have to end the food once you feel torment, disorder, and squeamishness. Most likely, this detoxification diet can have an enormous impact on the advancement and support of a healthy lifestyle.

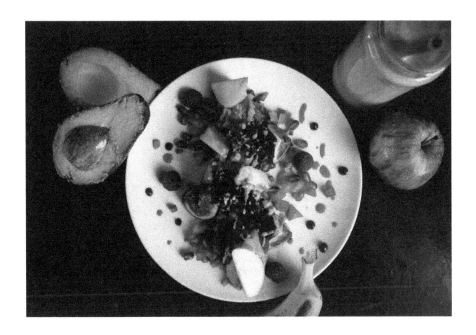

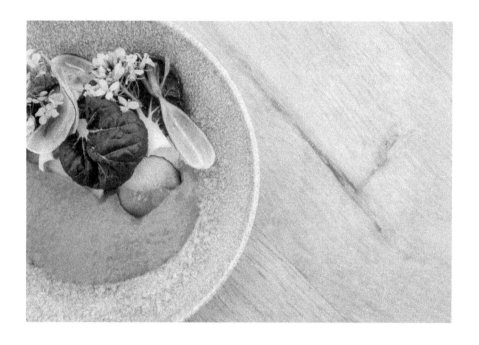

Chapter 3: Soups

1. Green Lentil Soup

Preparation Time: 10 minutes

Cooking Time: 30 minutes

Servings: 4

Ingredients:

- 1 ½ cups green lentils, rinsed
- 4 cups baby spinach
- 4 cups filtered alkaline water
- 1 tsp. Italian seasoning
- 2 tsp. fresh thyme
- 14 oz. tomatoes, diced
- 3 garlic cloves, minced
- 2 celery stalks, chopped
- 1 carrot, chopped
- 1 onion, chopped
- Pepper
- Sea salt

Directions:

1. Add all ingredients except spinach into the direct pot and mix fine.

2. Cover pot with top and cook on manual high pressure for 18 minutes.

3. When finished, release pressure using the quick release, and then open the lid.

4. Add spinach and stir well.

5. Serve and enjoy.

Nutrition:

- Calories 306
- Fat 1.5 g
- Carbohydrates 53.7 g
- Sugar 6.4 g
- Protein 21 g
- Cholesterol 1 mg

2. Squash Soup

Preparation Time: 10 minutes **Cooking Time:** 40 minutes

Servings: 4

Ingredients:

- 3 lbs. butternut squash, peeled and cubed
- 1 tbsp. curry powder
- 1/2 cup unsweetened coconut milk
- 3 cups filtered alkaline water
- 2 garlic cloves, minced
- 1 large onion, minced
- 1 tsp. olive oil

Directions:

1. Add olive oil in the instant pot and set the pot on sauté mode.
2. Add onion and cook until tender, about 8 minutes.
3. Add curry powder and garlic and sauté for a minute.
4. Add butternut squash, water, and salt and stir well.
5. Cover pot with lid and cook on soup mode for 30 minutes.
6. When finished, release pressure naturally for 10 minutes, then release using the quick release, and then open the lid.
7. Blend the soup utilizing a submersion blender until smooth.
8. Add coconut milk and stir well.
9. Serve warm and enjoy.

Nutrition:

- Calories 254 Fat 8.9 g Carbohydrates 46.4 g
- Sugar 10.1 g Protein 4.8 g Cholesterol 0 mg

3. Tomato Soup

Preparation Time: 5 minutes

Cooking Time: 20 minutes

Servings: 4

Ingredients:

- 6 tomatoes, chopped
- 1 onion, diced
- 14 oz. coconut milk
- 1 tsp. turmeric
- 1 tsp. garlic, minced
- 1/4 cup cilantro, chopped
- 1/2 tsp. cayenne pepper
- 1 tsp. ginger, minced
- 1/2 tsp. sea salt

Directions:

1. Add all ingredients to the direct pot and mix fine.
2. Cover the instant pot with a lid and cook on manual high pressure for 5 minutes.
3. When finished, release pressure naturally for 10 minutes then release using the quick release.
4. Blend the soup utilizing a submersion blender until smooth.
5. Stir well and serve.

Nutrition:

- Calories 81 Fat 3.5 g Carbohydrates 11.6 g
- Sugar 6.1 g Protein 2.5 g Cholesterol 0 mg

4. Basil Zucchini Soup

Preparation Time: 10 minutes

Cooking Time: 20 minutes

Servings: 4

Ingredients:

- 3 medium zucchinis, peeled and chopped
- 1/4 cup basil, chopped
- 1 large leek, chopped
- 3 cups filtered alkaline water
- 1 tbsp. lemon juice
- 3 tbsp. olive oil
- 2 tsp. sea salt

Directions:

1. Add 2 tbsp. oil into the pot and set the pot on sauté mode.
2. Add zucchini and sauté for 5 minutes.
3. Add basil and leeks and sauté for 2-3 minutes.
4. Add lemon juice, water, and salt. Stir well.
5. Cover pot with lid and cook on high pressure for 8 minutes.
6. When finished, release pressure naturally, then open the lid.
7. Blend the soup utilizing a submersion blender until smooth.
8. Top with remaining olive oil and serve.

Nutrition:

- Calories 157 Fat 11.9 g
- Carbohydrates 8.9 g Protein 5.8 g
- Sugar 4 g Cholesterol 0 mg

5. Summer Vegetable Soup

Preparation Time: 5 minutes **Cooking Time:** 20 minutes

Servings: 10

Ingredients:

- 1/2 cup basil, chopped
- 2 bell peppers, seeded and sliced
- 1/ cup green beans, trimmed and cut into pieces
- 8 cups filtered alkaline water
- 1 medium summer squash, sliced
- 1 medium zucchini, sliced
- 2 large tomatoes, sliced
- 1 small eggplant, sliced
- 6 garlic cloves, smashed
- 1 medium onion, diced
- Pepper
- Salt

Directions:

1. Combine all elements into the direct pot and mix fine.
2. Cover pot with lid and cook on soup mode for 10 minutes.
3. Release pressure using the quick release, then open the lid.
4. Blend the soup utilizing a submersion blender until smooth.
5. Serve and enjoy.

Nutrition:

- Calories 84 Fat 1.6 g Carbohydrates 12.8 g
- Protein 6.1 g Sugar 6.1 g Cholesterol 0 mg

6. Spicy Carrot Soup

Preparation Time: 10 minutes

Cooking Time: 20 minutes

Servings: 6

Ingredients:

- 8 large carrots, peeled and chopped
- 1 1/2 cups filtered alkaline water
- 14 oz. coconut milk
- 3 garlic cloves, peeled
- 1 tbsp. red curry paste
- 1/4 cup olive oil
- 1 onion, chopped
- Salt

Directions:

1. Combine all elements into the direct pot and mix fine.
2. Cover the pot with a lid, select the manual, and set the timer for 15 minutes.
3. Release pressure naturally, then open the lid.
4. Blend the soup utilizing a submersion blender until smooth.
5. Serve and enjoy.

Nutrition:

- Calories 267 Fat 22 g
- Carbohydrates 13 g Protein 4 g
- Sugar 5 g
- Cholesterol 20 mg

7. Zucchini Soup

Preparation Time: 10 minutes

Cooking Time: 30 minutes

Servings: 10

Ingredients:

- 10 cups zucchini, chopped
- 32 oz. filtered alkaline water
- 13.5 oz. coconut milk
- 1 tbsp. Thai curry paste

Directions:

1. Combine all elements into the direct pot and mix fine.
2. Cover pot with lid and cook on manual high pressure for 10 minutes.
3. Release pressure using the quick release, then open the lid.
4. Use a blender to blend the soup until smooth.
5. Serve and enjoy.

Nutrition:

- Calories 122
- Fat 9.8 g
- Carbohydrates 6.6 g
- Protein 4.1 g
- Sugar 3.6 g
- Cholesterol 0 mg

Chapter 4: Salads

8. Super-Seedy Salad with Tahini Dressing

Preparation Time: 10 minutes

Cooking Time: 0 minutes

Servings: 1-2

Ingredients:

- 1 slice stale sourdough, torn into chunks
- 50g mixed seeds
- 1 tsp. cumin seeds
- 1 tsp. coriander seeds
- 50g baby kale
- 75g long-stemmed broccoli, blanched for a few minutes then roughly chopped
- ½ red onion, thinly sliced
- 100g cherry tomatoes, halved
- ½ a small bunch flat-leaf parsley, torn

DRESSING

- 100ml natural yogurt
- 1 tbsp. tahini
- 1 lemon, juiced

Directions:

1. Heat the oven to 200°C/fan 180°C/gas 6. Put the bread into a food processor and pulse into very rough breadcrumbs. Put into a bowl with the mixed seeds and spices, season, and spray well

with oil. Tip onto a non-stick baking tray and roast for 15-20 minutes, stirring and tossing regularly, until deep golden brown.

2. Whisk together the dressing ingredients, some seasoning, and a splash of water in a large bowl. Tip the baby kale, broccoli, red onion, cherry tomatoes, and flat-leaf parsley into the dressing, and mix well. Divide between 2 plates and top with the crispy breadcrumbs and seeds.

Nutrition:

- Calories: 78
- Carbohydrates: 6 g
- Fat: 2g
- Protein: 1.5g

9. Sebi's Vegetable Salad

Preparation Time: 10 minutes

Cooking Time: 0 minutes

Servings: 1-2

Ingredients:

- 4 cups each of raw spinach and romaine lettuce
- 2 cups each of cherry tomatoes, sliced cucumber, chopped baby carrots and chopped red, orange and yellow bell pepper
- 1 cup each of chopped broccoli, sliced yellow squash, zucchini and cauliflower.

Directions:

1. Just wash all these vegetables. Mix in a large mixing bowl and top off with a non-fat or low-fat dressing of your choice.

Nutrition:

- Calories: 48
- Carbohydrates: 11g
- Protein: 3g

10. Greek Salad

Preparation Time: 10 minutes

Cooking Time: 0 minutes

Servings: 1-2

Ingredients:

- 1 Romaine head, torn in bits
- 1 cucumber sliced
- 1-pint cherry tomatoes, halved
- 1 green pepper, thinly sliced
- 1 onion sliced into rings
- 1 cup kalamata olives
- 1 ½ cups feta cheese, crumbled

For dressing combine:

- 1 cup olive oil
- 1/4 cup lemon juice
- 2 tsp. oregano
- Salt and pepper

Directions:

1. Layer ingredients on a plate. Drizzle dressing over salad.

Nutrition:

- Calories: 107
- Carbohydrates: 18g
- Fat: 1.2 g
- Protein: 1g

Chapter 5: Main Dishes

11. Sweet and Sour Onions

Preparation Time: 10 minutes

Cooking Time: 11 minutes

Servings: 4

Ingredients:

- 4 large onions, halved
- 2 garlic cloves, crushed
- 3 cups vegetable stock
- 1 ½ tablespoon balsamic vinegar
- ½ teaspoon Dijon mustard
- 1 tablespoon sugar

Directions:

1. Combine onions and garlic in a pan. Fry for 3 minutes, or till softened.
2. Pour stock, vinegar, Dijon mustard, and sugar. Bring to a boil.
3. Reduce heat. Cover and let the combination simmer for 10 minutes.
4. Get rid of from heat. Continue stirring until the liquid is reduced and the onions are brown. Serve.

Nutrition:

- Calories 203 Total Fat 41.2 gSaturated Fat 0.8 gCholesterol 0 mg Sodium 861 mgTotal Carbs 29.5 g
- Fiber 16.3 g Sugar 29.3 g Protein 19.2 g

12. Sautéed Apples and Onions

Preparation Time: 14 minutes

Cooking Time: 16 minutes

Servings: 3

Ingredients:

- 2 cups dry cider
- 1 large onion, halved
- 2 cups vegetable stock
- 4 apples, sliced into wedges
- A pinch of salt
- A pinch of pepper

Directions:

1. Combine cider and onion in a saucepan. Bring to a boil until the onions are cooked and liquid is almost gone.
2. Pour the stock and the apples. Season with salt and pepper. Stir occasionally. Cook for about 10 minutes or until the apples are tender but not mushy. Serve.

Nutrition:

- Calories 343 Total Fat 51.2 g
- Saturated Fat 0.8 g Cholesterol 0 mg
- Sodium 861 mg
- Total Carbs 22.5 g
- Fiber 6.3 g
- Sugar 2.3 g
- Protein 9.2 g

13. Zucchini Noodles with Portabella Mushrooms

Preparation Time: 14 minutes

Cooking Time: 16 minutes

Servings: 3

Ingredients:

- 1 zucchini, processed into spaghetti-like noodles
- 3 garlic cloves, minced
- 2 white onions, thinly sliced
- 1 thumb-sized ginger, julienned
- 1 lb. chicken thighs
- 1 lb. portabella mushrooms, sliced into thick slivers
- 2 cups chicken stock
- 3 cups of water
- A pinch of sea salt, add more if needed
- A pinch of black pepper, add more if needed
- 2 tsp. sesame oil
- 4 tbsp. coconut oil, divided
- ¼ cup fresh chives, minced, for garnish

Directions:

1. Pour 2 tablespoons of coconut oil into a large saucepan. Fry mushroom slivers in batches for 5 minutes or until seared brown. Set aside. Transfer these to a plate.

2. Sauté the onion, garlic, and ginger for 3 minutes or until tender. Add in chicken thighs, cooked mushrooms, chicken stock, water, salt, and pepper stir mixture well. Bring to a boil.

3. Decrease gradually the heat and allow simmering for 20 minutes or until the chicken is forking tender. Tip in sesame oil.

4. Serve by placing an equal amount of zucchini noodles into bowls. Ladle soup and garnish with chives.

Nutrition:

- Calories 163
- Total Fat 4.2 g
- Saturated Fat 0.8 g
- Cholesterol 0 mg
- Sodium 861 mg
- Total Carbs 22.5 g
- Fiber 6.3 g
- Sugar 2.3 g
- Protein 9.2 g

14. Grilled Tempeh with Pineapple

Preparation Time: 12 minutes

Cooking Time: 16 minutes

Servings: 3

Ingredients:

- 10 oz. tempeh, sliced
- 1 red bell pepper, quartered
- 1/4 pineapple, sliced into rings
- 6 oz. green beans
- 1 tbsp. coconut aminos
- 2 1/2 tbsp. orange juice, freshly squeeze
- 1 1/2 tbsp. lemon juice, freshly squeezed
- 1 tbsp. extra virgin olive oil
- 1/4 cup hoisin sauce

Directions:

1. Blend the olive oil, orange and lemon juices, coconut aminos or soy sauce, and hoisin sauce in a bowl. Add the diced tempeh and set aside.

2. Heat up the grill or place a grill pan over medium-high flame. Once hot, lift the marinated tempeh from the bowl with a pair of tongs and transfer them to the grill or pan.

3. Grill for 2 to 3 minutes, or until browned all over.

4. Grill the sliced pineapples alongside the tempeh, then transfer them directly onto the serving platter.

5. Place the grilled tempeh beside the grilled pineapple and cover

with aluminium foil to keep warm.

6. Meanwhile, place the green beans and bell peppers in a bowl and add just enough of the marinade to coat.

7. Prepare the grill pan and add the vegetables. Grill until fork tender and slightly charred.

8. Transfer the grilled vegetables to the serving platter and arrange artfully with the tempeh and pineapple. Serve at once.

Nutrition:

- Calories 163
- Total Fat 4.2 g
- Saturated Fat 0.8 g
- Cholesterol 0 mg
- Sodium 861 mg
- Total Carbs 22.5 g
- Fiber 6.3 g
- Sugar 2.3 g
- Protein 9.2 g

15. Courgettes in Cider Sauce

Preparation Time: 13 minutes **Cooking Time:** 17 minutes

Servings: 3

Ingredients:

- 2 cups baby courgettes
- 3 tablespoons vegetable stock
- 2 tablespoons apple cider vinegar
- 1 tablespoon light brown sugar
- 4 spring onions, finely sliced
- 1 piece of fresh ginger root, grated
- 1 teaspoon of corn flour
- 2 teaspoons of water

Directions:

- Bring a pan with salted water to a boil. Add courgettes. Bring to a boil for 5 minutes. Meanwhile, in a pan, combine vegetable stock, apple cider vinegar, brown sugar, onions, ginger root, lemon juice and rind, and orange juice and rind. Take to a boil. Lower the heat and allow simmering for 3 minutes. Mix the corn flour with water. Stir well. Pour into the sauce. Continue stirring until the sauce thickens.
- Drain courgettes. Transfer to the serving dish. Spoon over the sauce. Toss to coat courgettes. Serve.

Nutrition:

- Calories 173 Total Fat 9.2 g Saturated Fat 0.8 g Cholesterol 0 mg Sodium 861 mg Total Carbs 22.5 g Fiber 6.3 g Sugar 2.3 g
- Protein 9.2 g

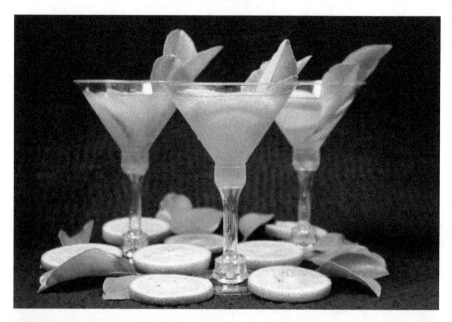

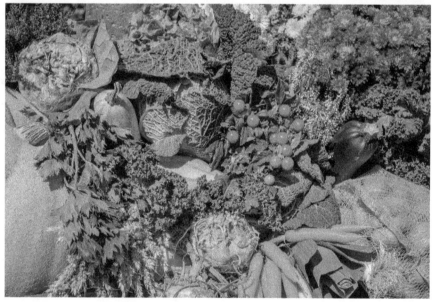

Chapter 6: Alkaline Diet Recipes to Get Rid of Herpes

16. Kale Pesto Pasta

There is no better way to eat your green than by making this cool kale pesto pasta. Make sure to try at your home for lunch.

Preparation time: 15 minutes

Cooking time: 12 minutes

Servings: 1

Ingredients:

- 1/2 cup walnuts
- 1 bunch kale
- 2 cups basil, fresh
- 1/4 cup oil
- 2 limes, freshly squeezed
- Salt and pepper
- 1 zucchini, spiralized
- Asparagus, cherry tomatoes, and spinach leaves for garnish

Directions:

1. Soak the walnuts overnight.
2. Add the walnuts with all other ingredients except the zucchini

in a food processor and pulse until well blended.

3. Add the zucchini mix and serve garnished with asparagus, cherry tomatoes and spinach. Enjoy.

Nutrition:

- Calories: 176
- Total fat: 17g
- Saturated fat: 3g
- Net carbohydrates: 5g
- Protein: 4g
- Fiber: 1g
- Sodium: 314mg

17. Spinach With Chickpeas and Lemon

If looking for an alkaline lunch to carry in your lunch box as part of a busy lifestyle, this flavorful easy recipe is the one for you.

Preparation time: 5 minute

Cooking time: 10 minutes

Servings: 2

Ingredients:

- 3 tablespoons oil
- 1 onion, thinly sliced
- 4 garlic cloves, minced
- 1 tablespoons ginger, grated
- 1/2 container cherry tomatoes
- 1 lemon, freshly zested and juiced
- 1 tablespoon red pepper flakes, crushed
- 1 can chickpeas
- Salt to taste

Directions:

1. Add oil in a skillet and cook onions until browned. Add garlic cloves, ginger, tomatoes, zest, and pepper flakes. Cook for 4 minutes.

2. Add chickpeas and cook for 3 more minutes. Add spinach and

cook until they start to wilt.

3. Add lemon juice and season with salt to taste. Cook for 2 more minutes.

4. Serve and enjoy.

Nutrition:

- Calories: 209
- Total fat: 8.1g
- Saturated fat: 1g
- Total carbohydrates: 28.5g
- Protein: 22.5g
- Fiber: 6g
- Sodium: 372mg
- Potassium: 286mg

18. Raw Green Veggie Soup

A delightful and welcoming flavorsome soup that is completely energizing and uplifting especially during Dr. Sebi's diet.

Preparation time: 5 minutes

Cooking time: 5 minutes

Servings: 1

Ingredients:

- 1 avocado
- 1 zucchini, chopped
- 2 celery stalks, chopped
- 2 cups spinach
- 1/4 cup parsley, fresh
- 2 sliced green peppers
- 1/8 onion, chopped
- 1 garlic clove
- 1/4 cup almonds, soak overnight, and rinse
- Salt to taste
- 1-1/2 cup water
- 1 lemon juice
- Diced watermelon radish for garnish

Directions:

1. Add all the ingredients in a food processor except salt.
2. Pulse until smooth or until the desired consistency is desired.
3. Pour the soup in a saucepan to warm a little bit before seasoning with salt and squeezed lemon.
4. Garnish with watermelon radish and enjoy.

Nutrition:

- Calories: 48.9
- Total fat: 0.4g
- Saturated fat: 0.1g
- Total carbs: 10.6g
- Net carbs: 6.7g
- Protein: 3.1g
- Sugars: 1.9g
- Fiber: 3.9g
- Sodium: 619mg
- Potassium: 417mg

19. Kale Caesar Salad

An easy and classic way to enjoy your kale during lunchtime. The dish is filling and complements Dr. Sebi's diet.

Preparation time: 5 minutes

Cooking time: 12 minutes

Servings: 1

Ingredients:

- 1 bunch of curly kale, washed
- 1 cup sunflower seeds
- 1/3 cup almond nuts
- 1/8 tablespoon chipotle powder
- 2 garlic cloves
- 1-1/4 water
- 1-1/2 tablespoon agave syrup
- 1/2 tablespoon sea salt

Directions:

1. Wash and pat dry the curly kale and remove the center membrane .tear the kale leaves into small sizes.
2. Add all other ingredients in a blender and blend until smooth and creamy.
3. Pour half of the mixture over the kale and toss until well coated.

4. Pour the remaining mixture and mix until the kales are well coated on the curls and folds.

5. Let rest for 10 minutes then serve on plates. Sprinkle sunflower seeds and enjoy.

Nutrition:

- Calories: 157
- Total fat: 6g
- Saturated fat: 2g
- Total carbohydrates: 18g
- Protein: 9g
- Sugars: 1g
- Fiber: 2g
- Sodium: 356mg

20. Red and White Salad

The macadamia nuts and avocado oil add a beautiful buttery flavor to this salad. You can also use your favorite nuts and oil.

Preparation 5 minutes **Cooking:** 10 minutes **Servings:** 2

Ingredients:

- 3 radishes
- 1 fennel bulb, greens removed
- 1/2 jicama, peeled and halved
- 2 celery stalks
- Juice from 1 lime
- 1/4 cup avocado oil
- Salt to taste
- Macadamia nuts

Directions:

1. Slice radish, fennel, jicama, and celery using a mandolin slicer on the thinnest setting. Toss them in a mixing bowl with lime and oil. Season with salt then top with nuts.

Nutrition:

- Calories: 197 Total fat: 9g Saturated fat: 4g Total carbs: 20g
- Protein: 7g Sugars: 1g Fiber: 2g Sodium: 366mg

21. Almond Milk

This is an awesome alternative to cow milk that is healthy, cheap, and very easy to make. Serve the milk with your favorite alkaline side for a filling lunch.

Preparation time: 5 minutes **Cooking time:** 10 minutes

Servings: 2

Ingredients:

- 1.7oz almonds, sliced
- 133.8 oz filtered water
- 1 tablespoon sunflower granules
- 2 dates, stones removed

Directions:

1. Soak the almonds for a few hours ahead of time.
2. Add all the ingredients in a blender and blend for 2 minutes.
3. Pour the milk in a container through a straining cloth. Carry in your lunch box or store in a fridge for up to 3 days.
4. You can use almond pulp in cakes or almond mixes.

Nutrition:

- Calories 90 Total fat: 2.5g Total carbohydrates: 16g
- Protein: 1g Sugars: 4g Sodium: 140mg Potassium: 140mg

22. Creamy Kale Salad With Avocado and Tomato

This alkaline bowl is healthy, delicious, and filling. It's also very easy to assemble and can be carried to work in your lunchbox.

Preparation time: 5 minutes

Cooking time: 10 minutes

Servings: 2

Ingredients:

- 2 handful of kale
- 2 cherry tomatoes
- 1 ripe avocado
- Juice from 1 lime
- 1 garlic clove, crushed
- 1 tablespoon agave
- 1/2 tablespoon paprika
- 1/2 tablespoon black pepper

Directions:

1. Wash kale and tomatoes and roughly chop them. Place them in a mixing bowl.
2. Peel the avocado and add it to the mixing bowl.
3. Add lemon juice and the rest of the ingredients to the bowl and

mix them thoroughly.

4. Serve and enjoy.

Nutrition:

- Calories: 179.2

- Total fat: 14.1g

- Saturated fat: 1.9g

- Total carbohydrates: 13.5g

- Protein: 3.7g

- Sugars: 6g

- Fiber: 6.1g

- Sodium: 77mg

- Potassium: 624mg

23. Creamy Broccoli Soup

This is a thick and flavorful soup recipe. It is simple quick and the most delicious soup to serve for lunch.

Preparation time: 5 minutes

Cooking time: 10 minutes

Servings: 5

Ingredients:

- 2 cups vegetable stock
- 4 cups broccoli, chopped
- 1 red pepper, chopped
- 1 avocado
- 2 onions, chopped
- 2 celery stalks, sliced
- Ginger to taste
- 1 tablespoon salt

Directions:

1. Warm vegetable stock in a small pot. Add broccoli and season with salt to taste. Simmer for 5 minutes.
2. Add the broccoli in a blender with pepper, avocado, onions, and celery stalks. Add some water for thinning then blend until smooth.

3. Serve when warm with ginger to your liking. Garnish with a lemon slice. Enjoy.

Nutrition:

- Calories: 270
- Total fat: 18g
- Saturated fat: 11g
- Total carbohydrates: 17g
- Protein: 12g
- Sugars: 5g
- Fiber: 3.5g
- Sodium: 470g

Chapter 7: Sauces

24. Sweet Barbecue Sauce

Preparation Time: 14 minutes

Cooking Time: 16 minutes

Servings: 3

Ingredients:

- 6 quartered plum tomatoes
- 1/4 cup of chopped white onions
- 1/4 cup of date sugar
- 2 teaspoons of pure sea salt
- 2 teaspoons agave syrup
- 1/4 teaspoon cayenne
- 2 teaspoons of onion powder
- 1/2 teaspoon ground ginger
- 1/8 teaspoon cloves

Directions:

1. Add all ingredients, excluding date sugar, to a blender and blend them thoroughly. Pour mixture into a saucepan and add a date sugar. Cook over average heat, stirring occasionally to prevent sticking until boiling. Reduce heat to a simmer. Cover the saucepan with a lid and cook for 15 minutes, stirring from time to time.

2. Use an immersion blender to blend the sauce until it is smooth.

Remain to cook at low heat until the sauce thickens for about 10 minutes. Allow mixture to cool before using it. Serve and enjoy your sweet barbecue sauce!

Nutrition:

- Calories: 30
- Carbohydrates: 4 g
- Fat: 1 g

25. Avocado Sauce

Preparation Time: 14 minutes

Cooking Time: 16 minutes

Servings: 3

Ingredients:

- 1 ripe avocado
- 1 pinch of basil
- ½ teaspoon of oregano
- 1/2 teaspoon of onion powder
- 2 teaspoons of minced onion
- 1/2 teaspoon of pure sea salt

Directions:

1. Cut the avocado in half, peel it and remove the seed. Slice it into small pieces and throw into a food processor. Add all other ingredients and blend for 2 to 3 minutes until smooth. Serve and enjoy your avocado sauce!

Nutrition:

- Calories: 14
- Carbohydrates: 2 g
- Protein: 1g

26. Fragrant Tomato Sauce

Preparation Time: 14 minutes

Cooking Time: 16 minutes

Servings: 3

Ingredients:

- 5 Roma tomatoes
- 1 pinch of basil
- 1 teaspoon of oregano
- 1 teaspoon of onion powder
- 2 teaspoon of minced onion
- 2 teaspoon agave syrup
- 1 teaspoon of pure sea salt
- 2 tablespoons of grape seed oil

Directions:

1. Make an X cut on the lowermost of the Roma tomatoes and place them into a pot of hot water for just 1 minute. Take away the tomatoes from the water using a spoon and shock them, placing them in cold water for 30 seconds. Take them out and immediately peel with your fingers or a knife. Put all the ingredients into a mixer or a food processor and blend for 1 minute until smooth. Serve and enjoy your fragrant tomato sauce.

Nutrition:

- Calories: 20 Carbohydrates: 2 g Protein: 1g

Chapter 8: Special Ingredients

27. Aquafaba

Preparation Time: 15 minutes

Cooking Time: 2 Hours 30 Minutes

Servings: 2-4 Cups

Ingredients:

- 1 bag of garbanzo beans
- 1 teaspoon of pure sea salt
- 6 cups of spring water + extra for soaking

Directions:

1. Place garbanzo beans in a large pot, add spring water and pure sea salt. Bring to a rolling boil.
2. Remove from the heat and leave to soak kindly for 30 to 40 minutes.
3. Strain garbanzo beans and add 6 cups of spring water.
4. Boil for 1 hour and 30 minutes on medium heat.
5. Strain the garbanzo beans. This strained water is Aquafaba.
6. Pour Aquafaba into a glass jar with a lid and place it into the refrigerator.
7. After cooling, Aquafaba becomes thicker. If it is too liquid, repeatedly boil for 10-20 minutes.

Useful tips:

- Aquafaba is a good alternative for an egg:

- 2 tablespoons of Aquafaba = 1 egg white

- 3 tablespoons of Aquafaba = 1 egg.

Nutrition:

- Calories: 46

- Carbs: 8 g

- Fiber: 2 g

- Protein: 3 g

Chapter 9: Snacks & Bread

28. Sweet Potato Chips

Preparation Time: 5 minutes

Cooking Time: 5 minutes

Servings: 4

Ingredients:

- 1 sweet potato, thinly sliced
- 2 teaspoons olive oil, or as needed
- Coarse sea salt, to taste

Directions:

1. Toss sweet potato with oil and salt.
2. Spread the slices in a baking dish in a single layer.
3. Cook in a microwave for 5 minutes until golden brown.
4. Serve.

Nutrition:

- Calories 213
- Total Fat 8.5 g
- Saturated Fat 3.1 g
- Cholesterol 120 mg
- Sodium 497 mg
- Total Carbs 21.4 g
- Fiber 0 g
- Sugar 0 g
- Protein 0.1g

29. Chia Crackers

Preparation Time: 20 minutes

Cooking Time: 1 hour

Servings: 24-26 crackers

Ingredients:

- 1/2 cup of pecans, chopped
- 1/2 cup of chia seeds
- 1/2 teaspoon cayenne pepper
- 1 cup of water
- 1/4 cup of nutritional yeast
- 1/2 cup of pumpkin seeds
- 1/4 cup of ground flax
- Salt and pepper, to taste

Directions:

1. Mix around 1/2 cup chia seeds and 1 cup water. Keep it aside.
2. Take another bowl and combine all the remaining ingredients. Combine well and stir in the chia water mixture until you obtained dough.
3. Transfer the dough onto a baking sheet and rollout (¼" thick).
4. Transfer into a preheated oven at 325°F and bake for about half an hour.
5. Take out from the oven, flip over the dough, and cut it into desired cracker shape/squares.
6. Spread and back again for a further half an hour, or until crispy and browned.

7. Once done, take out from the oven and let them cool at room temperature. Enjoy!

Nutrition:

- 41 calories
- 3.1g fat
- 2g total carbohydrates
- 2g protein

30. Crispy Crunchy Hummus

Preparation Time: 10 minutes

Cooking Time: 10-15 minutes

Servings: 4

Ingredients:

- 1/2 a red onion
- 2 tablespoons fresh coriander
- 1/4 cup of cherry tomatoes
- 1/2 a red bell pepper
- 1 tablespoon dulse flakes
- Juice of lime
- Salt to taste
- 3 tablespoons olive oil
- 2 tablespoons tahini
- 1 cup of warm chickpeas

Directions:

- Prepare your Air Fryer cooking basket
- Add chickpeas to your cooking container and cook for 10-15 minutes, making a point to continue blending them every once in a while until they are altogether warmed
- Add warmed chickpeas to a bowl and include tahini, salt, lime
- Utilize a fork to pound chickpeas and fixings in glue until smooth
- Include hacked onion, cherry tomatoes, ringer pepper, dulse drops, and olive oil
- Blend well until consolidated

- Serve hummus with a couple of cuts of spelt bread

Nutrition:

- Calories: 95 kcal
- Carbohydrates: 5 g
- Fat: 5 g
- Protein: 5 g

31. Pita Chips

Preparation Time: 5 minutes

Cooking Time: 12 minutes

Servings: 4

Ingredients:

- 12 pita bread pockets, sliced into triangles
- 1/2 cup olive oil
- 1/2 teaspoon ground black pepper
- 1 teaspoon of garlic salt
- 1/2 teaspoon dried basil
- 1 teaspoon dried chervil

Directions:

1. Set your oven to 400 degrees F.
2. Toss pita with all the remaining ingredients in a bowl.
3. Spread the seasoned triangles on a baking sheet.
4. Bake for 7 minutes until golden brown.
5. Serve with your favourite hummus.

Nutrition:

- Calories 201 Total Fat 5.5 g
- Saturated Fat 2.1 g
- Cholesterol 10 mg
- Sodium 597 mg
- Total Carbs 2.4 g
- Fiber 0 g
- Sugar 0 g
- Protein 3.1g

32. Pumpkin Spice Crackers

Preparation Time: 10 minutes

Cooking Time: 60 minutes

Servings: 06

Ingredients:

- 1/3 cup of coconut flour
- 2 tablespoons pumpkin pie spice
- ¾ cup of sunflower seeds
- ¾ cup of flaxseed
- 1/3 cup of sesame seeds
- 1 tablespoon ground psyllium husk powder
- 1 teaspoon of sea salt
- 3 tablespoons coconut oil, melted
- 1 1/3 cups of alkaline water

Directions:

1. Set your oven to 300 degrees F.
2. Combine all dry ingredients in a bowl.
3. Add water and oil to the mixture and mix well.
4. Let the dough stay for 2 to 3 minutes.
5. Spread the dough evenly on a cookie sheet lined with parchment paper.
6. Bake for 30 minutes.
7. Reduce the oven heat to low and bake for another 30 minutes.
8. Crack the bread into bite-size pieces.

9. Serve

Nutrition:

- Calories 248
- Total Fat 15.7 g
- Saturated Fat 2.7 g
- Cholesterol 75 mg
- Sodium 94 mg
- Total Carbs 0.4 g
- Fiber 0g
- Sugar 0 g
- Protein 24.9 g

33. Spicy Roasted Nuts

Preparation Time: 10 minutes

Cooking Time: 15 minutes

Servings: 4

Ingredients:

- 8 oz. pecans or almonds or walnuts
- 1 teaspoon of sea salt
- 1 tablespoon of olive oil or coconut oil
- 1 teaspoon of ground cumin
- 1 teaspoon of paprika powder or chili powder

Directions:

1. Add all the ingredients to a skillet.
2. Roast the nuts until golden brown.
3. Serve and enjoy.

Nutrition:

- Calories 287
- Total Fat 29.5 g
- Saturated Fat 3 g
- Cholesterol 0 mg
- Total Carbs 5.9 g
- Sugar 1.4g
- Fiber 4.3 g
- Sodium 388 mg
- Protein 4.2 g

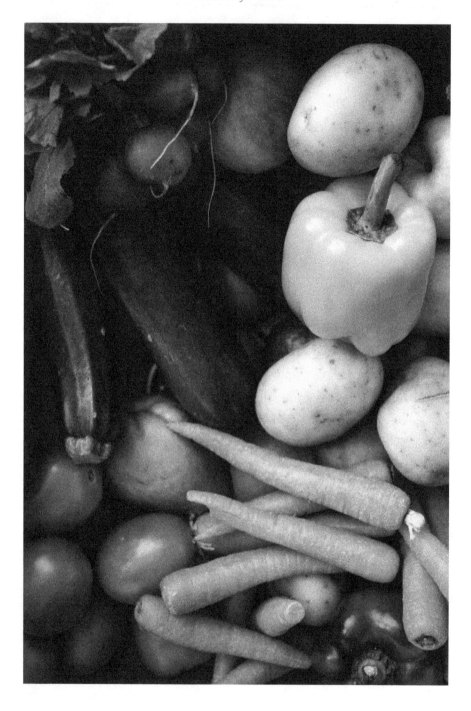

Chapter 10: Desserts

34. Blueberry Muffins

Preparation Time: 5 minutes

Cooking Time: 1 Hour

Servings: 3

Ingredients:

- 1/2 cup of blueberries
- 3/4 cup of teff flour
- 3/4 cup of spelt flour
- 1/3 cup of agave syrup
- 1/2 teaspoon of pure sea salt
- 1 cup of coconut milk
- 1/4 cup of sea moss gel (optional, check information)
- Grape Seed Oil

Directions:

1. Preheat your oven to 365 degrees Fahrenheit.
2. Grease or line 6 standard muffin cups.
3. Add Teff, Spelt flour, Pure Sea Salt, Coconut Milk, Sea Moss Gel, and Agave Syrup to a large bowl. Mix them together.
4. Add Blueberries to the mixture and mix well.
5. Divide muffin batter among the 6 muffin cups.
6. Bake for 30 minutes until golden brown.

7. Serve and enjoy your Blueberry Muffins!

Nutrition:

- Calories: 65

- Fat: 0.7 g

- Carbohydrates: 12 g

- Protein: 1.4 g

- Fiber: 5 g

35. Banana Strawberry Ice Cream

Preparation Time: 5 minutes

Cooking Time: 4 hours

Servings: 5

Ingredients:

- 1 cup of strawberry*
- 5 quartered baby bananas*
- 1/2 avocado, chopped
- 1 tablespoon of agave syrup
- 1/4 cup of homemade walnut milk

Directions:

1. Mix ingredients into the blender and blend them well.
2. Taste. If it is too thick, add extra milk or agave syrup if you want it sweeter.
3. Put in a container with a lid and allow to freeze for at least 5 to 6 hours.
4. Serve it and enjoy your banana strawberry ice cream!

Nutrition:

- Calories: 200
- Fat: 0.5 g
- Carbohydrates: 44 g

36. Homemade Whipped Cream

Preparation Time: 5 minutes

Cooking Time: 10 minutes

Servings: 1 Cup

Ingredients:

- 1 cup of Aquafaba
- 1/4 cup of agave syrup

Directions:

1. Add agave syrup and Aquafaba into a bowl.
2. Mix at high speed around 5 minutes with a stand mixer or 10 to 15 minutes with a hand mixer.
3. Serve and enjoy your homemade whipped cream!

Nutrition:

- Calories: 21
- Fat: 0g
- Sodium: 0.3g
- Carbohydrates: 5.3g
- Fiber: 0g
- Sugars: 4.7g
- Protein: 0g

37. "Chocolate" Pudding

Preparation Time: 5 minutes

Cooking Time: 20 minutes

Servings: 4

Ingredients:

- 1 to 2 cups of black sapote
- 1/4 cup of agave syrup
- 1/2 cup of soaked Brazil nuts (overnight or for at least 3 hours)
- 1 tablespoon of hemp seeds
- 1/2 cup of spring water

Directions:

1. Cut 1 to 2 cups of black sapote in half.
2. Remove all seeds. You should have 1 full cup of de-seeded fruit.
3. Mix all ingredients into a blender and blend until smooth.
4. Serve and enjoy your "chocolate" pudding!

Nutrition:

- Calories: 134
- Fat: 0.5 g
- Carbohydrates: 15 g
- Protein: 2.5 g
- Fiber: 10 g

38. gBanana Nut Muffins

Preparation Time: 5 minutes

Cooking Time: 1 Hour

Servings: 6

Ingredients:

Dry ingredients:

- 1 1/2 cups of spelt or teff flour
- 1/2 teaspoon of pure sea salt
- 3/4 cup of date syrup

Wet ingredients:

- 2 medium blended burro bananas
- ¼ cup of grape seed oil
- ¾ cup of homemade walnut milk (see recipe)*
- 1 tablespoon of key lime juice

Filling ingredients:

- ½ cup of chopped walnuts (plus extra for decorating)
- 1 chopped burro banana

Directions:

1. Preheat your oven to 400 degrees Fahrenheit.
2. Take a muffin tray and grease 12 cups or line with cupcake liners.

3. Put all dry ingredients in a large bowl and mix them thoroughly.

4. Add all wet ingredients to a separate, smaller bowl and mix well with blended bananas.

5. Mix ingredients from the two bowls in one large container. Be careful not to over mix.

6. Add the filling ingredients and fold in gently.

7. Pour muffin batter into the 12 prepared muffin cups and garnish with a couple of Walnuts.

8. Bake it for 22 to 26 minutes until golden brown.

9. Allow cooling for 10 minutes.

10. Serve and enjoy your banana nut muffins!

Nutrition:

- Calories: 150
- Fat: 10 g
- Carbohydrates: 30 g
- Protein: 2.4 g
- Fiber: 2 g

39. Mango Nut Cheesecake

Cooking Time: 4 Hour 30 Minutes

Servings: 8 Servings

Ingredients:

Filling:

- 2 cups of Brazil nuts
- 5 to 6 dates
- 1 tablespoon of sea moss gel (check information)
- 1/4 cup of agave syrup
- 1/4 teaspoon of pure sea salt
- 2 tablespoons of lime juice
- 1 1/2 cups of homemade walnut milk (see recipe)*

Crust:

- 1 1/2 cups of quartered dates
- 1/4 cup of agave syrup
- 1 1/2 cups of coconut flakes
- 1/4 teaspoon of pure sea salt

Toppings:

- Sliced mango
- Sliced strawberries

Directions:

- Put all crust ingredients in a food processor and blend for 30 seconds.

- With parchment paper, cover a baking form and spread out the blended crust ingredients.

- Put sliced mango across the crust and freeze for 10 minutes.

- Mix all filling ingredients using a blender until it becomes smooth.

- Pour the filling above the crust, cover with foil or parchment paper, and let it stand for about 3 to 4 hours in the refrigerator.

- Take out from the baking form and garnish with toppings.

- Serve and enjoy your mango nut cheesecake!

40. Blackberry Jam

Preparation Time: 5 minutes **Cooking Time:** 4 hours 30 minutes

Servings: 1 cup

Ingredients:

- 3/4 cup of blackberries
- 1 tablespoon of key lime juice
- 3 tablespoons of agave syrup
- ¼ cup of sea moss gel + extra 2 tablespoons (check information)

Directions:

1. Put rinsed blackberries into a medium pot and cook on medium heat. Stir blackberries until liquid appears.
2. Once berries soften, use your immersion blender to chop up any large pieces. If you don't have a blender put the mixture in a food processor, mix it well, then return to the pot.
3. Add sea moss gel, key lime juice, and agave syrup to the blended mixture. Boil on medium heat and stir well until it becomes thick.
4. Remove from the heat and leave it to cool for 10 minutes.
5. Serve it with bread pieces or the Flatbread (see recipe).
6. Enjoy your blackberry jam!

Nutrition:

- Calories: 43 Fat: 0.5 g Carbohydrates: 13 g

41. Blackberry Bars

Preparation Time: 5 minutes

Cooking Time: 1 hour 20 minutes

Servings: 4

Ingredients:

- 3 burro bananas or 4 baby bananas
- 1 cup of spelt flour
- 2 cups of quinoa flakes
- 1/4 cup of agave syrup
- 1/4 teaspoon of pure sea salt
- 1/2 cup of grape seed oil
- 1 cup of prepared blackberry jam

Directions:

1. Preheat your oven to 350 degrees Fahrenheit.
2. Remove the skin of the bananas and mash with a fork in a large bowl.
3. Combine agave syrup and grape seed oil with the blend and mix well.
4. Add spelt flour and quinoa flakes. Knead the dough until it becomes sticky to your fingers.
5. Cover a 9x9-inch baking pan with parchment paper.
6. Take 2/3 of the dough and smooth it out over the parchment pan with your fingers.

7. Spread blackberry jam over the dough.

8. Crumble the remaining dough and sprinkle on the top.

9. Bake for 20 minutes.

10. Remove from the oven and let it cool for at 10 to 15 minutes.

11. Cut into small pieces.

12. Serve and enjoy your blackberry bars!

Nutrition:

- Calories: 43

- Fat: 0.5 g

- Carbohydrates: 10 g

- Protein: 1.4 g

- Fiber: 5 g

Chapter 11: Smoothies

42. Apple Smoothie

Preparation Time: 15 minutes

Cooking Time: 0

Servings: 2

Ingredients:

- 2 cups of apple juice, fresh
- 2 cups ice cube
- 1 tbsp. sea moss
- 1 clove, grounded
- 1 tbsp. ginger, grounded

Directions:

1. To start with, place all the ingredients needed to make the smoothie in a high-speed blender. Blend all ingredients wait for 2 to 3 minutes or until you get a smooth mixture.
2. Serve and enjoy.

Nutrition:

- Calories: 431.5
- Fat: 10.8g
- Carbohydrates: 53.1g
- Protein: 38.4g

43. Weight Loss Apple Cucumber Smoothie

Preparation Time: 15 minutes

Cooking Time: 0

Servings: 1

Ingredients:

- One large to medium size of sliced cucumber
- One large cubed apple
- One large sliced bell pepper
- Six seeded dates (rinsed)
- Six large strawberries
- Five sliced tomatoes (rinsed)
- Half to one cupful of water

Directions:

1. Combine the whole recipes and blend very well until smooth. Wow! The first-day breakfast is settled, enjoy.

Nutrition:

- 65 calories
- Carb 57 g
- Protein 2 g
- Fat 4 g

44. Toxins Removal Smoothie

Preparation Time: 15 minutes

Cooking Time: 0

Servings: 1

Ingredients:

- One seeded and sliced small to large-sized watermelon
- One large key lime (removes the juice and discards the seed
- One large cucumber (sliced)

Directions:

1. Transfer the lime juice into the blender.
2. Add the remaining recipes and blend very well to obtain a smooth mixture.
3. Wow! This means you have successfully completed the second-day smoothie. Enjoy.

Nutrition:

- 45 calories
- Carb 35 g
- Protein 6 g
- Fat 4 g

45. Multiple Berries Smoothie

Preparation Time: 15 minutes

Cooking Time: 0

Servings: 1

Ingredients:

- A quarter cupful of blueberries
- A quarter cupful of strawberries
- A quarter cupful of raspberries
- One large banana (peeled and sliced)
- Agave syrup as desired
- A half cupful of water

Directions:

1. Transfer the water into the blender.
2. Add the remaining recipes and blend until smooth.
3. I really love this smoothie because it is very sweet without adding sugar and the colour is also inviting.

Nutrition:

- Calories: 210
- Carbohydrates: 55 g
- Sodium: 20 mg

46. Dandelion Avocado Smoothie

Preparation Time: 15 minutes

Cooking Time: 0

Servings: 1

Ingredients:

- One cup of dandelion
- One orange (juiced)
- Coconut water
- One avocado
- One key lime (juice)

Directions:

1. In a high-speed blend all ingredients until smooth.

Nutrition:

- Calories: 160
- Fat: 15 grams
- Carbohydrates: 9 grams
- Protein: 2 grams

47. Amaranth Greens and Avocado Smoothie

Preparation Time: 15 minutes

Cooking Time: 0

Servings: 1

Ingredients:

- One key lime (juice)
- Two sliced apples (seeded)
- Half avocado
- Two cups of amaranth greens
- Two cups of watercress
- One cup of water

Directions:

1. Add the whole recipes together and transfer them into the blender. Blend thoroughly until smooth.

Nutrition:

- Calories: 160
- Fat: 15 grams
- Carbohydrates: 9 grams
- Protein: 2 grams

48. Lettuce, Orange and Banana Smoothie

Preparation Time: 15 minutes

Cooking Time: 0

Servings: 1

Ingredients:

- One and a half cupsful of fresh lettuce
- One large banana
- One cup of mixed berries of your choice
- One juiced orange

Directions:

1. First, add the orange juice to your blender.
2. Add the remaining recipes and blend thoroughly.
3. Enjoy the rest of your day.

Nutrition:

- Calories: 252.1
- Protein: 4.1 g

49. Delicious Elderberry Smoothie

Preparation Time: 15 minutes

Cooking Time: 0

Servings: 1

Ingredients:

- One cupful of elderberry
- One cupful of cucumber
- One large apple
- A quarter cupful of water

Directions:

1. Add the whole recipes together into a blender. Grind very well until they are uniformly smooth and enjoy.

Nutrition:

- Calories: 106
- Carbohydrates: 26.68

50. Peaches Zucchini Smoothie

Preparation Time: 15 minutes

Cooking Time: 0

Servings: 1

Ingredients:

- A half cupful of squash
- A half cupful of peaches
- A quarter cupful of coconut water
- A half cupful of Zucchini

Directions:

1. Add the whole recipes together into a blender and blend until smooth and serve.

Nutrition:

- 55 Calories
- 0g Fat
- 2g Protein
- 10mg Sodium
- 14g Carbohydrate
- 2g Fiber

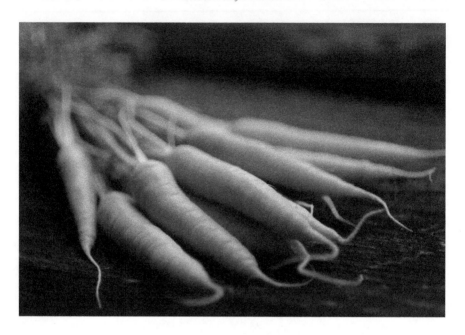

Conclusion

Thank you for making it to the end of Dr. Sebi's book of recipes. Dr. Sebi's eating regimen is an antacid dinner plan, which is generally a veggie lover diet. The eating regimen depends on plants that control human-made weight control plans and cross breed nourishments as well. The eating regimen likewise guarantees that there are least degrees of corrosive in the nourishments you devour and the bodily fluid in one's body.

He additionally accepts that when individuals follow the two strategies, they make a domain, basic, not perfect for the endurance of maladies in the human body.

What inspired the specialist to receive the eating regimen is his starting point back in Honduras. The inspiration driving Dr. Sebi's eating routine focuses back to Alfredo Darrington Bowman (Dr. Sebi). He is a local Honduran, known as an intracellular specialist, botanist, and common healer.

Eating food is an everyday schedule that people should experience. The idea of substances and nourishments that we devour ordinary can bring about a lifetime utilization propensity on the off chance that it isn't directed. Before hopping into the basic way of life, you have to contemplate it. It will assist you with abstaining from making void vows to self.

This eating routine diminishes body contaminants and supports general prosperity. It will make you take a more secure, better way to deal with food.

It will likewise raise the odds of different infections. On the chance that you need to shed pounds, it can spur you to do it effectively and dependably. This is identified with improved quality and versatility that everybody requires.

Dr. Sebi's eating regimen is an altogether new way to deal with food. Thusly, it may be difficult to become acclimated to it, particularly toward the beginning.

It is prudent to attempt Dr. Sebi's Directions for 30 days if you don't completely receive another dietary system. Connect with for a month and see the upgrades. Following a month, you should change to this eating regimen altogether.

Dr. Sebi's diet advances eating entire, natural, plant-based food. Numerous people have used to cause a noteworthy change in their wellbeing. They are perfect in moving from acidic to soluble. You can similarly utilize them for occasionally keeping up your body framework and improving your wellbeing.

Not exclusively will you eat scrumptious suppers, you will likewise be helping yourself and your family to feel much improved and improve in general wellbeing just by eating affirmed Doctor Sebi's food. How incredible is that?

Now there is just one thing for you to do: Take action!

I hope you enjoyed reading this book. If you are looking to follow a more plant-based eating pattern, Dr. Sebi's diet has many healthy diets that are more flexible and sustainable.

I wish you great success in your journey for good health!

CPSIA information can be obtained
at www.ICGtesting.com
Printed in the USA
BVHW080227020321
601389BV00003B/522

9 781914 167942